BOUNCE BACK

RECLAIM YOUR LIFE
AFTER A CONCUSSION

VANESSA WOODBURN

ISBN: 978-19-5-036772-6

Published by

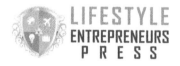

If you are interested in publishing through Lifestyle
Entrepreneurs Press, write to:
Publishing@LifestyleEntrepreneursPress.com

Publications or foreign rights acquisition of our catalog books.
Learn More: *www.LifestyleEntrepreneursPress.com*

Printed in the USA

On Eagle's Wings
I dedicate this book to my parents, Terry and Peggy.
You are both free now. On eagle's wings.
I promise to find my wings and fly,
knowing you are both there to raise me up.

CONTENTS

1

WILL THIS EVER GET BETTER?

You are holding this book because you or someone you love has experienced a concussion. Life feels like a rollercoaster right now, full of ups and downs and just as dizzying. Concussions can be compared to a *software* injury in the brain. Your *hardware* is intact, and on the outside, it appears as though everything is normal. "You look fine," people say. But on the inside, it feels as though everything has changed. Nothing is normal. It is the last thing you think about when you fall asleep and the first thing you think about when you wake up. You don't feel like yourself anymore.

People say you should be grateful that your incident wasn't more serious. You *are* grateful because you know this could have been worse. But it doesn't change the fact that your brain, this amazing, complex, miraculous system between your ears, has been impacted by a force that caused a firestorm in its cells. You have suffered a traumatic brain injury. Among so many other symptoms, you wonder, "How will I get through today? Will this headache last forever? Will I always be this tired and irritable? Will I remember everything I need to remember today? Will I be able to hold on and work out all the details in my head about this project? How is this affecting my family? Who am I now? Will this ever get better?"

Maybe the healing and recovery are happening along the timeline that your doctor gave you when you received your diagnosis. But perhaps your symptoms are lingering and you are still struggling long after you expected to feel like yourself again. You have days you begin to feel confident and capable again, but then you get slammed with random reminders that everything is not okay. Maybe it's in the form of a vice grip sensation in your head from morning until night, or a day when you feel dizzy and close to tears as you walk through the grocery store. It may be the way you startle so easily now, the buzzing and piercing heat that randomly storms through your brain, or the to-do list on your phone that sets off a flood of indecision.

Your family is experiencing this concussion as well. They can't feel your physical pain, but they sense your frustration and sadness. You feel guilty about how your injury affects them, the things you cannot do right now, the time and resources that your healing is taking, and the way you have changed as you try to cope with and manage your responsibilities at home and work. "They have no idea how hard I'm working to make this look easy," I sobbed to one of my healthcare providers about three months after my concussion. I didn't want my family to see me struggling. I wanted so badly to be okay and for them not to worry about me. I wanted my children to have their mother back.

The pretending is exhausting and lonely. You feel isolated as you go through this experience because it seems so hard to explain your challenges to people about how things are different for you now. Neurologically healthy people try to relate by saying things like, "Oh, I forget things all the time. Don't worry about that!" But those comments actually minimize the experience that you are living through and make you feel lonelier and more isolated. No one else knows the extent of what has changed, what now requires so much energy while making it look easy like you do.

Six months after my concussion I decided to attend a conference for health coaches in New York City. I had traveled solo dozens of times in my life, but this time I was terrified. I remember lying in bed the night before, crying, "What if I forget where to go? What if I get confused? What if I panic? What if I just don't know what to do?" My husband consoled and encouraged me, but it was impossible to explain to him the fear that felt so real behind these tears. I simply could not trust my brain to know, do, navigate, decide, and solve the things that had always felt easy and effortless. I'm certain that every single person I encountered in the airport and at that conference, saw a capable woman, but they had no idea of the effort and energy it required on my part to make that look easy.

The "what-ifs" after a concussion can keep you up at night. "What if I had done that differently? What if I had seen a different doctor afterwards, or rested more, or rested less? What if I am doing too much, or not enough? *What if this never gets better?*"

You believe that if nothing changes and you always feel stuck here, that the cost may be higher than you can bear. It affects every part of your life: relationships, career, happiness, sense of peace and safety, and sense of self. *Who am I now?* This is a quest to return to yourself, get back on your feet, feel healthy and whole, and recover a feeling of normalcy again for you and your family.

On my quest for healing, I began to learn that it was possible to change many of the thoughts and stories that were driving my fears about staying stuck. I began to learn about concussions and what I could do to take care of my body, my brain, and my emotional health after my trauma. I gradually learned that it was possible to rewire my brain to choose thoughts and feelings that honored the possibility and potential of my healing, rather than choosing stories based in fear. I began to see how much I was loved and supported. I learned to ask for help and even more importantly, how to receive it.

You have this book because you or someone you love has had a concussion. You also have this book because you believe in possibility and potential. So do I. I am honored to guide you through these steps to bounce back and reclaim your life.

2

THE ITALIAN BREAK – MY STORY

n 2016, my husband Oliver and I decided to do something grand to celebrate our twentieth wedding anniversary. So, we decided to join some friends of ours on a five-day bike tour through the gorgeous Italian region of Piedmont. I had done some road cycling and short distance triathlons early in my twenties, but around that time, my cycling experience involved riding around the parks and paths in our neighborhood with my kids. "No problem," I thought! I updated my gear with new cycling shoes and padded shorts and found a fantastic spin class at my local gym to condition myself.

The trip was booked for September 2016. Our children were ten, twelve, and fourteen at the time, so leaving them to go on vacation at the beginning of the school year was a difficult choice for me. Our son Noah would also be celebrating his thirteenth birthday while we were away. Oliver's sister and her husband agreed to move into our house for the week with their two young girls to hold down the fort so that we could enjoy this time away.

Oliver and I arrived in Turin, Italy, on September 16th. We met up with family, Tim and Sara, and we had a day to tour this beautiful city before meeting our cycling guides and the rest of the small group who we would be cycling with, including my childhood friend Karen and her husband Rob. Karen and I had traveled and adventured together as teenagers, but this was our first trip together in years! If you're a parent of young children, you know that time away from the kids, as a couple, is extra precious. I felt so good, free, and grateful to be able to get away like this with Oliver.

I'm not going to lie, the first day of cycling was *hard*. The rolling hills of Piedmont and medieval cobblestone villages, while stunning, were a challenge for a novice cyclist like me. But on day two I started to get more comfortable and confident, and began to enjoy the gorgeous scenery and countryside. When I woke up on day three of our tour, the first thing I thought about was our family at home and Noah's birthday, which they would be celebrating that day. Our group made plans to stop at the mid-way point in our day to film a *happy birthday!* video to send him.

That morning started crisp and cool. I remember having breakfast at the villa where we were staying and then setting off for the day with our group. I was happy and feeling good. We stopped for a road-side snack break around 10 a.m. and then set off down a long switchback descent. I remember the snacks, the view atop that hill, and enjoying the company of Karen and Sara as the three of us set off together at the rear of the group.

That is where my memories end. I am told that I navigated the switchback descent like a champ, slow and steady. The route then opened up into a fast, flat stretch, and I am told that this is where something went wrong. Perhaps it was a cramp in my hand that caused me to unexpectedly trigger the brake? Perhaps a moment of inattention? We will never know. Whatever the cause, I crashed on that flat stretch of road – hard, tumbling over and over. Sara was behind me and saw the whole thing. She managed to avoid crashing into me and was with me in seconds.

I was tangled in my bike, conscious, but very obviously confused. My helmet was cracked and there was a deep gash above my right eye. My knees, elbows, forearms, and hands were bloody. I have no memory of any of this and rely on the retelling of it by Sara, and then Karen, who was alerted by a passing motorist as to what had happened behind her and who rushed back.

I have only very brief flashbacks of moments of the twenty-four hours that followed my crash. I am told everyone immediately suspected a concussion, or worse, as I had obvious short-term memory loss and confusion. Although I knew the names of my children, I no longer remembered it was Noah's birthday. Our cycling guides got to me soon after the crash and had the training to assess, support, and direct the situation. We were in a rural area and it took some time for the ambulance to arrive. One of our guides who spoke Italian, along with Oliver and Karen, came with me in the ambulance and we drove, sirens wailing, to a hospital in a small town called Alba.

I spent the rest of that day being x-rayed, CT-scanned, cleaned, stitched, poked, and prodded – I have no memory of any of it. Oliver was with me through most of that day and he still marvels at how calm I was. He says I was conscious and did not seem to be in pain, scared, or upset.

My first stream of post-crash memories begins in a quiet, dimly-lit hospital room in the early hours of the next morning.

7

All the tests were done, the doctors were gone, and it was just Oliver and I. I think it felt safe for me at this point to wake up and begin storing memories again. I remember the light in the room, Oliver's gentle smile, and his reassurance that I was going to be okay. I had a concussion, liver trauma, and a fractured sternum, rib, and cheekbone, but I was going to be okay. "She will recover," the doctors had told Oliver, but due to the laceration and bruising in my liver, I would need to stay in this Italian hospital on bedrest for days, maybe weeks, or longer. The hardest and most shocking thing to hear was that we would have to stay in Italy and be separated from our children for such a long time.

I realized that the crisis was over, but the journey was just beginning.

We talked via video call with our family at home every day. It was so hard being halfway across the world and separated from each other. Life continued at home in the capable hands of my sister and brother-in-law – school, carpool, band, music lessons, playdates for my younger two, and a memorable first date for my almost-fifteen-year-old.

As for me, my Italian adventure continued. These days in the hospital were hard for so many reasons; I did not speak Italian and many of the doctors and nurses did not speak English. We often had to rely on Google Translate, which was awful for medical jargon to the point of being laughable. I had terrible headaches, my body ached all over, and for the first time in my life, I experienced frequent anxiety and panic attacks. These would usually come on in the middle of the night and since I had no experience with this, I had no idea how to control them. Through tears, I would try to communicate my fear and racing heartbeat to the nurses, who did not understand me, which would increase my sense of panic. I now understand that this experience is common after a brain injury and trauma, but at the time, it was all new.

Looking back, this time in the hospital began to teach me about the power of trust and surrender. I had very little control over the situation, especially given the lack of communication and understanding of how I was healing. I needed to trust that the people around me were caring, qualified professionals. The doctors had a plan, I was slowly getting better, and we had to trust them. My job during this time was to rest and let my body begin healing.

My concussion symptoms were all over the map. I remember crushing headaches, feeling very emotional, hot flashes that would leave me soaking wet, being extremely sensitive to noise, having difficulty sleeping, dizziness, and feelings of panic and anxiety, mostly at night.

After about ten days, the doctors agreed that I could leave the hospital, but I was not allowed to go very far. Oliver found a ground-floor flat to rent just down the street from the hospital in Alba. I was still not allowed to fly home, and this seemed like a good "halfway house" for us. I have very peaceful, tender memories of these days. It was as if I knew that it would be the calm before the storm. We enjoyed slow walks around town and morning coffees in the market square. My physical symptoms slowly began to improve. Oliver even rented a car one day and we drove to a few of the places we missed on the bike tour.

I was finally given the all-clear to fly home on October 3rd, a few days before the Canadian Thanksgiving holiday. The reunion with our family at home was so sweet. We had been away for three weeks. I remember the kids wanting to hug me but being afraid to hurt me. I remember cuddling on the couch with my daughter and marveling at her compassion and empathy as she asked, "Were you scared, Mommy? Did it hurt? Did they take care of you?" I am eternally grateful for the force of love and the circle of friends and family that surrounded our children during that time to make sure that they felt loved, safe, and cared for.

It was not until we were home and I was trying to get back into some kind of normal routine that I began to realize the full extent of my concussion symptoms. I often felt dizzy, anxious, teary, and irritable for what seemed like no good reason. Simple, everyday things would completely trip me up, like starting to unload the dishwasher and then not remembering where to put things, trying to return permission forms and pizza orders for the kids' schools but having no idea how to break down these tasks to complete them. Picking up a book to read, and having to read and re-read over and again to understand the content. Bumping into familiar people in the store and coming up against a blank wall when I tried to remember their names. Going out to do the grocery shopping at my regular store and lacking the ability to pull up a map in my head of where things were or how they might be categorized.

I have always been a good student. I love learning. I loved school. I was smart and got excellent grades. My friends joked about my almost-photographic memory. I had always relied on my intellect as my superpower. And now, more than any other system in my body, my concussion affected what is called *executive function* in my brain – higher-order cognitive tasks like memory, decision making, organizing, and prioritizing. This was a huge blow to my confidence and made me feel like I had lost the old me. My familiar ways of navigating the world were gone. I could not count on my brain to do things that had always felt easy and natural. I began writing in my journal during this time and would ask myself questions like, "Who am I now? The old me is gone. Everything feels different."

Around six weeks after my accident, my family doctor told me that I was "fine." He had run the neurological tests that doctors are trained to do and there were no red flags. He felt there was nothing more he could do to help me. This terrified me because I knew that I was not fine. I was not *me*. I refused to believe that I would just have to sit back and wait for this to get better (or not) and decided it was time to become my own advocate and health coach, to seek a process, healers, helpers, and treatments that would help me get back on my feet.

I believe in an approach to health that considers the whole person – not just isolated symptoms, but the physical body as well as emotional and mental wellness. I don't know about your experiences, but I like the feeling of being seen and heard by a practitioner who takes the time to ask questions about how you are doing as a whole, and who listens and responds carefully to really get to the root of a problem.

I am not interested in treating symptoms without trying to understand why. So, I used this underlying belief as a guide as I searched for people who could help me. Once I found someone who I resonated with and experienced results with, I began to rely on their network for referrals. Gradually my multi-disciplinary healthcare team grew and I began to notice improvement in my symptoms, both physically and emotionally. This was never a linear path, and one of my greatest lessons has been learning how to manage my frustration and expectations through the up and down nature of recovery.

After a year or so, I began to feel capable and confident enough in my recovery to begin stepping out in a different way. I began reaching out to people, not as a patient, but as a health coach, sharing my story and helping others. I was trained through the Institute for Integrative Nutrition™ to help guide people on their wellness journey in a holistic, integrative way. It was the exact framework that I was using to help and heal myself through the healthcare I sought, the courses I took, the people I surrounded myself with, and the books I read.

Over time, I began to offer general talks and workshops for women who were interested in learning about this integrative approach to wellness. My own concussion symptoms continued to ease, and I was still actively working with a healthcare team to continue my progress. Two and a half years post-concussion, I decided that I was ready to begin offering my coaching and guidance to the concussion community and to both patients and caregivers. I felt called to focus my work more deeply within this community. I accepted several invitations to speak to support groups and women's groups to share my story of navigating this journey and what I was learning along the way about hope and healing.

My inspiration for writing this book was born from the experiences I have had and the people I have met through coaching, and in my talks and workshops over the past three years. I began to realize that in a world that so often focuses on the negative, people were yearning to hear from someone with a voice that is passionate, empowered, and hopeful about healing. These words from Dr. Joe Dispenza, author of *Breaking The Habit of*

Being Yourself, ring so very true: "The passion you have for your suffering, you have to have that for your healing." So, I wrote this book to share my passion for healing with you.

3

LAYING THE TRACKS
TO BOUNCE BACK

wrote this book as a guide to help people get back on their feet after a concussion. Our bodies have an amazing ability to heal and most people who experience a concussion will heal on their own within a week or two. However, I know from experience that if you are one of the unlucky ones whose concussion symptoms persist longer than fourteen days, then a diagnosis of post-concussion syndrome (PCS) can become a long, lonely, winding road. As of the time of writing this book, I am more than three years post-concussion. But now, through trial and error, finding skilled helpers as well as applying the knowledge, tools, and strategies that I learned from them, discovering my own positive and hopeful determination to heal, and yes, *time*, I have healed completely.

I was halfway through my certification at the Institute for Integrative Nutrition to earn my designation as a health coach when my accident happened. I was granted extra time to finish my coursework and I felt so grateful that I was able to apply much of what I was learning to my own health and healing. I also began to connect myself to a network of people to treat my symptoms. A physiotherapist, an osteopath, a chiropractor, a naturopath, and a therapist all helped me work through the roller coaster of emotions and feelings I was going through.

As an Integrative Nutrition Health Coach, I am the perfect person to guide and coach you on this path so you feel like you can bounce back and get your life back after a concussion. It is not within my scope of practice to diagnose a concussion or to treat your symptoms. I will, however, offer suggestions on where you can find qualified, experienced healthcare professionals who can. This book will also help you lay the tracks for your healing and support wherever you are on your journey and for you to begin to feel capable and confident even when your symptoms are persisting.

I have discovered that the stories we tell ourselves have great power over our thoughts and behavior. I will guide you through how to shift your language and your thoughts, as well as how to write a new story about your healing and potential that is positive and hopeful. When we do this work, there is always the possibility that we may uncover new strengths and skills. I will help you embrace the idea that there could be growth and more for you than you can imagine right now. You may want to keep a notebook or a journal nearby to write down ideas, suggestions, questions, or anything else that comes up for you as we go along. I suggest reading the chapters in order, as each one builds on the steps of the chapter before it. However, if something really sticks out for you, feel free to jump ahead!

I realize that everyone's journey through post-concussion is different. Every concussion and trauma is unique. Symptoms and their duration vary greatly from person to person, and also vary within each of us over time. The cost of staying in a place of struggling and suffering is great. It not only affects us, but also our families, friends, workplaces, and communities. What we all share is a desire to get back up, feel normal again, regain our sense of self after all this upheaval, and feel healthy and whole. I believe there is something here for you whether you are two months or two years or more on your journey, and that these steps may be exactly the guide that you are looking for.

This book introduces a seven-step process to guide you on how to reclaim your life after a concussion. Here's a brief outline of each of these seven steps:

Step One: **Understanding what happened to you and who can help.** Concussions are an invisible injury. A general understanding of the current theory and physiology of what happens when someone experiences a concussion is helpful. After all, knowledge is power.

Step Two: **Self-care after a concussion**. There are simple everyday things you can do at home to encourage healing. In this chapter, we'll discuss how to take care of yourself, body, mind, and spirit.

Step Three: **Ask for help and allow people to give it.** This is a time in your life when it's necessary to ask for help and, even more importantly, to receive the help and support that is offered. I will teach you how you can become more open to this and why it's important.

Step Four: **The love you give is for you too.** This chapter is about self-compassion, learning how to talk to yourself like someone you love, and why this is some of the most important work you will ever do.

Step Five: **Brave the valley.** In everyone's journey there comes a valley – a time of change where life can feel difficult and lonely. This chapter is about learning to walk bravely through your valley and to unearth the treasures it has to offer along the way.

Step Six: **Writing your own story.** Our brains are wired for stories and wired to keep us safe. In this chapter, you will learn how to choose thoughts and stories that are empowering, rather than stories that keep you feeling stuck and stagnant.

Step Seven: **You have permission to grow.** After making it through this upheaval in your life, you may find that you feel brand new in many ways. Learn how to embrace this change and evolution.

I believe that you can lean on this process to help guide you through your post-concussion journey and at other times in your life when you feel like things are falling apart at the seams. These steps now live in my bones and it is my honor to guide you through them.

4

WHAT HAPPENED AND WHO CAN HELP YOU?

Current statistics tell us that about 3.8 million Americans experience a concussion every year. The most common ways to sustain a concussion are from contact sports, falls, and motor-vehicle accidents. Many people I meet have a story about someone they know who has experienced a concussion. Dr. Cameron Marshall, founder of Complete Concussion Management, shares that most people feel "back to normal" within ten to fourteen days after injury, and usually make a full recovery within three to four weeks. For thirty to thirty-five percent of people, symptoms may linger, and about ten percent report persistent symptoms more than a year following their injury. Research on concussions is evolving rapidly and the vast majority of concussions are now viewed as treatable injuries that can be rehabilitated. If you are one of the people whose symptoms persist after the first week or so, the number one predictor of the speed of your recovery is how soon you see a concussion-care clinician.

As an Integrative Nutrition Health Coach, it is not within my scope of practice to diagnose or treat a concussion. My goal here is to increase your awareness, help you understand what a concussion is, and provide information about where you can look for help.

What Is a Concussion?

After my concussion, I often wondered what happened in my brain. I believe that knowledge is power and it was important for me to have some kind of understanding. According to the *Complete Concussion Management Handbook*, "A concussion is a form of brain injury that causes a temporary disturbance in how your brain functions. Concussions happen because of a hit, bump or blow to the head or elsewhere on the body. This impact causes the brain to move back and forth inside the skull."

The current theory is that a concussion is caused by the stretching and shearing of the brain cells that happens after a hit or blow to the head or the body. These stretching and shearing forces cause an electrical firestorm to occur in the brain, as ion channels open up and chemicals rush in and out of the brain cells. This firestorm, or "excitatory phase," in the brain may explain why people report "seeing stars," confusion, and memory loss. This phase is followed by an extreme drop in brain energy, as the brain works hard to restore the ion imbalance. Energy drops drastically during this crisis and begins to slowly rebuild and recover over the next few weeks. If you have had a concussion and experienced extreme fatigue in the days and weeks after, this can explain why.

If you are interested in learning more about the physiology of a concussion, check out the twelve minute "What Is a Concussion?" video by Dr. Cameron Marshall on YouTube.

Every concussion is different and symptoms vary. If you suspect you have a concussion, or have been diagnosed, immediately stop activity and see your doctor or a licensed healthcare provider for an assessment. They will check to make sure there are no red flags of a more serious injury, like skull fracture or brain bleed, and will discuss parameters for rest from school, work, or play. Refer to the *Complete Concussion Management Handbook*.

Who Can Help Treat Your Concussion Symptoms?

After I returned home from Italy, I went to see my family doctor. I shared with him all the reports from the hospital, and after some neurological tests in his office, he confirmed my concussion diagnosis. He told me to rest and come back in a week. When I returned a week later, about one-month post-concussion, we went through the battery of neurological tests again, assessing things like balance, visual disturbance, and working memory function, among others. The results? I was told to go home and return to my regular life as I felt able. I was self-employed at the time, so there were no criteria for returning to work that I had to meet.

For me, this is where a stark new reality began to set in. I was recovering, but also still experiencing physical, cognitive, and emotional symptoms. There were so many changes in how my brain was working, or not working, that were invisible to others, like my problem-solving, decision-making, and prioritizing abilities, as well as my memory. My family doctor had assessed that I was neurologically "intact," but we did not discuss how to actively treat, or rehabilitate, these lingering symptoms. At this point, I began to feel that my recovery and progress were up to me.

I began to reach out to my network of friends and colleagues in holistic healthcare to put together what would eventually become a multi-disciplinary team. I searched specifically for clinicians who had experience treating people with concussions. One of the first people I found was an osteopathic practitioner. This was a pivotal decision for me, as osteopathic treatments, including myofascial release and cranial sacral therapy, helped both my body and brain heal from the trauma I had experienced. Osteopathy was my first experience with a healthcare practice that addressed my body, mind and spirit as a whole, integrated system. This approach has been a very good fit for me. The practitioner who I saw was also well-connected in the healthcare community and he referred me to several other clinicians who offered effective treatments and therapies.

One of the first referrals he gave me was to a physiotherapist who practiced in a Complete Concussion Management (CCM) clinic. CCM clinics are run by rehab-based professionals such as physiotherapists, chiropractors, or athletic therapists who have undergone extensive training based on the most current, evidence-based research about rehabilitating people who have experienced concussions. They receive monthly research updates and must re-certify every two years. There are currently 350 active CCM Clinics worldwide, and there may be one in your community (https://completeconcussions.com/

services-courses/patients-athletes/). If you do not have access to a CCM clinic, look for practitioners who are open to a collaborative approach to your healing and who have a dedicated and reputable experience treating concussions. Many qualified professionals also have an online space where they offer support and current, evidence-based advice that you can access from home. I recommend Concussion Doc, Molly Parker PT, ConcussionCompass.com, and RehabLab.ca all of whom share valuable content online and on social media.

If you go to a CCM clinic, you will receive a thorough assessment, including a physical exam and questionnaire that addresses and tracks dozens of symptoms. A treatment and rehab plan will be prescribed, one tailored specifically for you that may include guided exercise therapy to help restore blood flow to your brain. Depending on the particular area of expertise of the clinic you choose, you may also receive manual therapy to address cervical (neck) issues, vestibular therapy for dizziness and balance, acupuncture, visual therapy, and emotional support and reassurance. You may be referred to a specialist for speech therapy, endocrinology, neuropsychology, or neuro-optometry, if necessary. This seems like an awfully long list, doesn't it? The reason why it takes such a collaborative and multi-disciplinary approach is that a concussion is a neurological injury for a short period of time. Once the acute phase is over, there can be a cascade of other effects that need rehabilitation and treatment.

Over my first few months post-concussion, my team grew to include osteopathy, physiotherapy, chiropractic care, naturopathy, massage therapy, and psychotherapy. Managing the appointments and treatments truly was my full-time job. I made a decision that if this was what it was going to take to get back on my feet, then it was worth my time, money, and energy. I used a paper calendar to keep track of all the appointments and a notebook to write down my questions, answers, treatment advice, and other things that I needed to remember.

Side-note: I was discharged from the first CCM clinic that I went to about eight months post-concussion. Two years later I experienced a return of significant dizziness and vision/vestibular issues, so I went back to a CCM clinic. Don't be afraid to return to a practitioner or clinic months (or years!) after your injury if you experience new or returning symptoms. Recovery from concussion is not linear. In my case, two months of acupuncture, at-home vestibular exercises, and manual cervical (neck) therapy resolved these issues.

I am pleased to hear that as the research around concussions grows, many in the field are beginning to embrace new, empowering language in how they label concussion symptoms. For example, the term *persistent concussion symptoms* is now often used in place of *post-concussion syndrome*. I agree with this shift because calling lingering symptoms *persistent*, rather than a *syndrome*, provides language and reassurance for patients and families that healing and recovery is possible. Persistent doesn't mean forever. It just means *right now* this is present, not this will *always* be present.

You are the only one who truly knows your body. Listen to it. If you need help, or wonder if your symptoms can be "fixed," no matter how long it has been, ask. Concussion-care is a growing field and there are more resources available now than there were just a few years ago. The field of concussion research and evidence-based treatment is constantly evolving.

If a practitioner recommends that you rest in a dark room, or use a "wait and see" approach, they are likely not up-to-date and you have the right to ask for a second opinion. Choose a collaborative, multi-disciplinary approach and look for rehab-based clinicians who are staying current with the science and knowledge needed to treat concussions.

5

SELF-CARE FOR YOUR BODY, MIND, AND SPIRIT

This chapter is about how to take care of yourself after a traumatic experience or event with self-care that goes beyond pedicures, bubble baths and bonbons. This is about learning how to nurture and nourish yourself, and understanding what you need while you are healing so that you can show up and reclaim your life. When you do this work to honor *yourself,* only then can you show up for the people who need and depend on you. This kind of deep self-care in the midst of the firestorm in your body, mind, and spirit after a trauma it is not always easy. But it may be the most important work you will ever do.

This work requires courage. It requires you to be brave and vulnerable and to ask of yourself, *What do I need? What will nourish me?* And I am not just referring to food as your only source of nourishment. When I talk about self-care, I mean your *whole* self. Your physical body needs care and nourishment, but so does your mind and your spirit. In this chapter, I will address self-care from this holistic perspective. I encourage you to take what you need from the list of self-care options that I suggest and leave the rest. You decide when it's the right timing and what is a good fit for you.

Our bodies are wise. They know what we need. The work is in learning to listen, and then acting on what we hear. This might be a new skill for you and may not feel easy at first. When your body is in survival mode, it will tell you. It may feel like butterflies in your stomach, a fluttering heart, quick shallow breaths, startling easily, or like you are living on the edge *all of the time*. When you get these messages from your body, listen.

This is the sympathetic branch of your autonomic nervous system on high alert, ready for fight, flight, or freeze. It is your body's survival mechanism and a natural response to trauma and stress. There are things you can do to help calm your nervous system and to communicate to your body that the emergency is over and that you are safe now. Doing so triggers the para-sympathetic branch of your nervous system to take over, which controls the rest, digest, and restore response in your body. Many of the self-care suggestions below can help to activate the parasympathetic system.

Yoga

Once you are cleared by your concussion-care team, find a gentle or restorative yoga class. A yoga practice can help you breathe and be present in your body in a way that supports the calming response you are looking for. You can gently stretch and move while honoring what you feel and what you need. Yoga can help release muscle tension in your body, promote self-awareness in your mind, and invite stillness and self-acceptance in your spirit. It is through yoga that I first began to develop an awareness of the emotions that I held in my body. I can still hear the voice of my first instructor, Robyn, saying, "Can you give yourself permission to just be here? With whatever you feel right now? No judgement. Just let it come and then let it go." She made it feel safe to do this. Gentle yoga can be a transformative practice for you to restore a sense of calm and balance in your body.

Meditation

Meditation is a practice that can help you calm the racing thoughts in your head and learn how to pay attention to your breath in a way that calms and restores your nervous system. It is priceless because it can become a tool that you carry with you always. As human beings, we *think* virtually all the time. If you have extra stress and anxiety in your life, this constant stream of thought leaves you with no respite, no inner peace.

Many yoga studios now offer mediation and mindfulness classes, or there are online resources if you prefer to learn on your own. There are also apps such as *Headspace, Calm,* and *Insight Timer.* An effective meditative tool to promote relaxation is a breathing exercise that I learned from Integrative M.D. Dr. Andrew Weil. It's called 4-7-8 breathing. Find a quiet space and sit on the edge of a chair with your feet planted on the ground, or you may prefer to lie down. Close your eyes and relax your shoulders. Breathe in through your nose for a count of four, hold for seven, then breathe out through your mouth for a count of eight. Repeat this three or four times. This simple practice is a great way of calming the nervous system when we start to feel anxious or have racing thoughts. It also gives the brain a new focus – breathing, instead of racing thoughts.

I went to see my family physician again about a year after my concussion. My thoughts were scattered, I was constantly worried and anxious about small things, and I was stressed about "not feeling like myself." I am grateful that my doctor recognized this was a big shift for me and a new pattern in my behavior, and that he wanted to help me learn how to change this. He referred me to a mindfulness-based stress reduction program (MBSRP), a twelve-week series of mindfulness meditation classes. This class was a deep dive into self-care for my mind, body, and spirit.

One of my favorite analogies to explain the benefits of mindfulness meditation comes from the book *Wherever You Go, There You Are* by Jon Kabat-Zinn. He relates our incessant stream of thoughts to a coursing river. We so often get caught up in the current of the river and this can end up carrying us to places we never planned to go. "Meditation means learning how to get out of the current, sit by its bank and listen to it, learn from it, and then use its energies to guide us rather than to tyrannize us." My a-ha moment from the MBSRP class was learning to find a pause in my thoughts. In this pause, we have the power to *choose* a response, rather than react in an automatic way. When you are seeking to reclaim your life and your thoughts after a concussion, this is a useful practice to learn.

Exercise and Movement

When we move our bodies, it encourages blood flow to the brain and through the body, which supports the healing process. This can also be a great way to heal and care for your body and your nervous system in a way that is calming and that requires you to listen. Listen to your body and what it is saying you need. You may have a treatment plan from a clinician telling you to exercise in a specific heart-rate zone to increase blood flow. So, listen to the professionals, but outside of your treatment plan, if you feel like movement, listen to your body. Ask yourself, "What do I need – a walk, yoga, a swim, something more, something less?" Allow yourself to be curious. Permit yourself to try something new and know that it's okay to change your mind if that doesn't feel good. I also find that just being outside, walking, while I take in fresh air and feel the ground beneath my feet is another effective way to nurture a feeling of calm.

Massage Therapy

A visit to a massage therapist can do wonders to help promote the feelings of rest and relaxation that your body is craving. All registered massage therapists will do a complete health history before they begin and you can let them know about your concussion, your general health, and how you are feeling on that day. Together, you can decide exactly what will be the most restorative and effective treatment for you, perhaps an aromatherapy, Swedish, or hot stone massage. Whatever you choose, enjoy!

Food and Nutrition

Nutrition plays such an important role in healing after trauma. I think of nutrition and the food we eat as information for our bodies and our cells. Our bodies want to be in balance, and food is a tool we can use to help our bodies heal. Inflammation is a common problem after concussion. We can help calm this response in our bodies by eating anti-inflammatory foods. Some of my favorites that I recommend include:

- leafy greens
- avocados
- wild blueberries
- ginger
- turmeric
- green tea
- wild-caught salmon
- healthy fats from fish oils, flax seed, and walnuts

Staying well-hydrated is also so important! Feel free to drink herbal teas or add a slice of lime or lemon to your water if it encourages you to consume more. Try for at least eight glasses of water a day.

There are several supplements that are currently being studied for their anti-inflammatory and possibly even neuroprotective benefits. Most of these are based on animal studies, but the supplements that show promising results with few risks or side effects at appropriate dosages are:

- Omega-3 – found in fish oil
- Curcumin – found in turmeric
- Resveratrol – found in the skin of red grapes, berries, and peanuts
- Vitamin C – found in broccoli, cantaloupe, kiwi, and citrus fruits
- Vitamin D3 – found in wild-caught salmon, egg yolks, and sunshine
- Creatine – found in meat and fish

The Gut-Brain Connection

The gut and brain are connected physically through the vagus nerve which stretches from the brain stem all the way down to the abdomen, and biochemically through neurotransmitters, which are chemicals produced in the brain and gut that control feelings and emotions. There is growing research that trauma to the gut or brain is co-related because of these physical and biochemical connections. We can help the gut-brain connection by stimulating the vagus nerve with simple interventions in many of the self-care suggestions mentioned above such as deep breathing, yoga, moderate exercise, meditation and massage therapy. The vagus nerve is a key player for the critical healing response to rest, digest and restore so any attempt to stimulate and balance its function is helpful. Another fun thing you can try is singing! Singing has been shown to have a biologically soothing effect, connected to the vagus nerve.

Chemically, we can help the gut-brain connection by eating anti-inflammatory foods and foods that contain probiotics and prebiotics which promote healthy bacteria and microbes in the gut, such as:

- Omega-3 fats from flax seed or fish oil
- Fermented foods such as sauerkraut, miso, kimchi, and yogurt
- High-fiber foods like nuts, seeds, fruits, and vegetables

A naturopathic doctor or functional medicine specialist can help to tailor a personalized plan for you to strengthen your gut health. This may include food sensitivity testing to learn which foods may be irritating and inflammatory for you. Eliminating these foods from your diet for an eight to twelve-week trial period can be a very effective way to reduce inflammation in your body and restore your gut health.

Sleep

A good sleep routine is a critical component of your self-care after a concussion because sleep helps the brain recover and clear inflammation. Sleep disturbances post-concussion, however, are common. You may find that you have trouble falling asleep or staying asleep. Try to keep to your normal bedtime schedule every night, even on the weekends. If you have trouble falling asleep, get up and do something relaxing until you feel sleepy and then try again. If you feel tired during the day, set a timer and allow yourself a fifteen-minute nap so it does not affect the restorative sleep that your body and brain need at night.

Your concussion-care team may suggest supplementing with melatonin. You may also want to try a meditation app such as *Calm* or *Insight Timer*, which have guided meditations or music that can help with sleep. There is also new science that shows that thirty minutes of blue light *in the morning* can have a positive effect on our circadian rhythm (our body's sleep/wake cycle that is critical for healing after a concussion). People who were exposed to thirty minutes of blue light after waking were able to fall asleep faster and had better quality sleep. We do get blue light from screens, but if you're interested in trying this suggestion, I recommend a blue light lamp on a timer for thirty minutes in the morning.

What to Avoid After a Concussion

Now that we have discussed the self-care tips that are helpful post-concussion, there are a few things that are definitely *not* helpful and should be avoided.

- Avoid added sugar, alcohol, and highly-processed foods in your diet. These contribute to inflammation in your brain and in your body. Many naturopaths also recommend avoiding gluten and dairy products, as they can have an inflammatory effect.
- Limit your screen use. Screens are like strobe lights flashing into your brain, which can be overwhelming input during a time when your brain is already in an energy deficit.
- The advice to shut yourself away in a dark room is now considered outdated and unhelpful for two reasons – one, your brain needs light during the day and gentle stimulation after a concussion, and two, isolating yourself this way is not helpful for your emotional health.
- Avoid returning to school, work, activities, or sports until you have been cleared by your healthcare provider.

Get Creative

Creativity can be a healing place to channel your thoughts and emotions after a traumatic experience. Maybe you already have a creative practice that feels like the right place to play with this. If you don't, allow yourself to be curious. Would some type of art or music feel good?

After my accident, I started to notice that every time I heard an acoustic song on the radio my ears perked up. I would often start to cry when I heard stripped-down versions of songs. But these weren't tears of suffering, they were healing tears. So, I listened to more of this type of coffeehouse-style of music. Then I decided to dust off a guitar that was sitting in my basement. I took my guitar to a few local music studios to ask about lessons and interview teachers.

Important note here – I was very honest with them. I was two months post-concussion. My brain felt like a fuzzy mess. I knew that this wasn't going to be an easy thing to learn and I let my teacher know that I was struggling with cognitive tasks. I knew, however, that there was something about playing the guitar that my body and my spirit needed – the exercise for my brain, the vibration of the strings on my chest, the sounds washing into my ears.

I eventually found the perfect teacher for me and committed to lessons. It was a very slow process at first, but I know that it was an important part of my healing on so many levels. It was rarely easy, but I always knew that it was healing work. I encourage you to explore your creative side. Allow yourself to play with this idea and whatever you come up with that feels right for you. It may be just the thing to nurture and nourish your brain, body, and spirit!

Seek Connection

Another important aspect of self-care is spending time with the people who can hold a safe place for you to just be you. Seek out friends who can bear the weight of your struggles, who can listen and witness how you are feeling, and with whom you can also share good times, fun, and laughter. Friends and loved ones can help you find that balance which you may need if you find that you are isolating yourself. If your feelings, emotions, or struggles are taking over your life, an important part of self-care also includes finding a therapist, counselor, or group that you feel comfortable talking to in order to take care of your emotional and mental health.

My best advice to nurture your self-care after a concussion is to take care of your mind, body, and spirit in all the ways I have shared above:

- eat healthy whole food
- get good sleep
- drink lots of water
- enjoy sunlight and fresh air
- find quiet and stillness through yoga and meditation
- exercise and move your body
- enjoy hugs and talks with friends and loved ones
- laugh
- make time for activities that get your creative juices flowing, that you enjoy, and that feel fun.

Discovering what you need to truly nurture and nourish yourself at this time is important work. Your healing is worthy of the time and effort it takes to begin to build this practice of self-care for your body, mind, and spirit.

6

HELP – IT'S TIME TO ASK AND RECEIVE

When did we first hear the message, *the rule*, that asking for help shows weakness or that it puts an unfair burden on the people you are asking? I heard this somewhere in my childhood and young adult life. So, when the biggest crisis of my life occurred, I had the opportunity to look at this rule and decide for myself if I was going to live by it or not. I learned that when life presents you with a crisis, a fall, a loss, or a heartbreak, you can choose to go it alone or you can choose to surrender and trust that there are people around you who can help, who want to help, and that humbly *receiving* their help can be a gift to both of you.

As I mentioned, one of the most important healing things you can do to care for yourself after a traumatic event is to ask for what you need. This may often mean asking for help, especially after a concussion, when even the simplest tasks can be a challenge. If you have grown up with the programming that asking for help shows weakness or puts an unfair burden on others, this may be a big step for you.

Asking For Help

There is research on resilience and our ability to "bounce back" after crisis that shows that of all the learned skills and tools that people can apply in the face of trauma, it is the resources around us that most help us get back on our feet. Our network of friends, colleagues, and family certainly counts as a resource. Asking for help means learning to be aware of how you are feeling, what you need, and reaching out to ask for help, knowing that it is one of the bravest and most effective ways to move forward in your healing and recovery.

This was one of my first lessons after my concussion. I became aware of it daily. My daughter's eleventh birthday party was one of my first big challenges when we got home from Italy. I was six weeks post-concussion and my party planning and organizing skills were non-existent. I was sad that planning this party for her was so hard for me. It showed me, clear as day, all the things that I could not do. All the ways that I believed I was "less than." It aggravated my grief and feelings of loss.

As her birthday got closer, I decided to ask for help, rather than try to push through. I explained to my husband that this task, with all its moving parts, felt overwhelming and created a kind of *cognitive fatigue* for me that was exhausting. It seemed silly. What's so hard about planning a kid's birthday party? But asking for help was actually a breakthrough for me because it gave me a chance to be honest with my family about how I was struggling. Remember my comment in chapter one – "They don't know how hard I'm working to make this look easy?" Here was a chance for me to show my family where I needed help, to show them what wasn't easy.

My husband very capably and enthusiastically took over as chief party planner. Together with our sons, who were thirteen and fifteen years old at the time, he threw an unforgettable "Hollywood Game Night" party for our girl. For the first time in my life, I sat back and just watched my daughter's birthday party unfold. I vividly remember the laughter and joy in the room. Everyone had fun, including me! It was a lesson for me to give myself permission to surrender, ask for help, and allow treasures to appear in unexpected places.

After an unexpected event like a concussion, you may find that help shows up for you in many different ways and at different times. It may be meals delivered to your house, or people offering to do the logistical things like buy groceries, drive you to appointments, clean your house, invite your kids over to play, or do your carpool drives. Help may also come in the days and weeks after the initial crisis is over. It looks like hugs that speak volumes when there are no words that can touch your suffering, friends who check in often, especially when they notice that you have become very quiet, and people who reach out for a coffee date, days and months later. Help looks like people who can just be with you and listen because sometimes we can't fix these things.

Help will also come from clinicians in the multi-disciplinary teams who know how to treat your symptoms and help you continue moving toward your full recovery. For me, reaching out to a therapist to ask for help after my concussion was a big step forward in learning about the strength required to take care of myself and to ask for help. I love these words from author Jen Hatmaker in her book *Of Mess And Moxie*: "There is nothing weak about being in the care of a counselor. That is strong, sister. That says you are not passively waiting for your strength, your restoration. You are doing the work, poking the bear...It is a sign of incredible strength."

Receiving Help

In the days in the hospital following my accident, Oliver and I had our first lesson in the power of allowing ourselves to receive help. Family who were with us on this trip had plane tickets booked to continue their vacation in London, England, for a few days after the bike tour in Italy. When we all learned that I was not going to be discharged from the hospital for days or weeks, Tim and Sara offered to cancel their tickets and stay with us. At first, Oliver refused. This seemed so unfair and burdened them with extra costs and arrangements. Thankfully, Tim was able to help Oliver understand that they wanted, they needed, to stay with us, even if only for a few days. I think those five days that the four of us spent together ended up being a very special memory for each of us in our way.

Oliver had someone to lean on for support and logistics as he worked to find accommodations and form a plan for our unexpected stay. Sara ran errands around Alba for me to find little things like toiletries and comfy clothes that I needed. I'll never forget her helping me wash my hair in the hospital. We made such a mess and giggled through the whole process. We would later learn from Tim and Sara that being able to stay and help us both was exactly the therapy they needed to soothe their worried and broken hearts. That was my first lesson in the power of *receiving* help that people offer – it can also be a gift for them. Somehow, we were able to help them heal from the shock of the accident by gratefully accepting their help, love, and support.

Isn't it beautiful that we are all designed with different strengths so that we can show up for each other, each in our unique way, and offer our unique gifts at just the right time? I worked with a client once who struggled to ask for help, and even when it was offered freely to her, she was reluctant to receive it. We discussed all the ways that she lived a generous life and how much she loved helping her friends and family. I helped her see that this was now a chance to let the circle flow and gratefully receive the love and support from others that she gave so willingly. She had spent her whole life loving, supporting, helping, and giving. This was the garden she had cultivated, and now it was okay, it was *good*, to reap what she had sowed with a grateful and humble heart.

Give yourself permission to receive the help that is offered to you and I promise, it will help you discover what your superpowers are. You will know how it feels to be on the receiving end and you will become the perfect person to help others when their time of need comes along. It becomes a circle that continues to generate more of the things that really matter in life – love, gratitude, joy, giving, and receiving. Difficult times and challenges happen for all of us at some point. When your friends or family need *you*, you may find that your ability to listen, show compassion, and offer your gifts might feel like the most natural thing in the world, because you know how it feels to be on the receiving end. It is not a burden for us to be there for each other. It is how we are designed – to be in community and connection with one another.

7

THE LOVE YOU GIVE IS FOR YOU TOO

"Can you talk to yourself like you talk to someone you love?" were the words my therapist spoke to me in the darkest days of my concussion recovery. Those days were dark because months after my accident, there were still whispered comments like, "Are you still struggling? Maybe you're just lazy. Are you even trying? You fell off a bike. That's it! Why is this taking so long?!"

These comments were crushing.

Crushing because the person saying all this was *me*. That was *my* voice in my head, my thoughts in my journal. I wrote these journal entries in capital letters, yelling at myself.

This was the point in my recovery when, thankfully, I was introduced to the concept of self-compassion, of talking to myself like I talk to someone I love. I understood compassion. I had received it from my friends and my family. I knew how to be a compassionate person with my children, husband, friends, and even strangers. I did not, however, know how to offer it to myself. The therapist I was seeing walked me through this by saying, "If your daughter came home from school after a really difficult day feeling sad and discouraged, how would you talk to her?"

I said, "I would give her a hug. I would find out what she needs. I would just be with her and love her."

"Yes," she said. "Can you be with yourself that way? Can you talk to yourself that way, love yourself that way?"

This was the beginning of a radical change in my life. I gradually began to understand that *the love I give to others is for me too*. In my moments of sadness, frustration, and discouragement, my work was to love myself through it, to be compassionate with myself, to understand that I can also offer myself the love I so freely give to others. I needed to talk to myself like I talk to a loved one.

Dr. Kristin Neff and Dr. Christopher Germer are at the forefront of research on self-compassion, which is now garnering more and more attention. In Dr. Neff's words, "Instead of mercilessly judging and criticizing yourself for various inadequacies or shortcomings, self-compassion means you are kind and understanding when confronted with personal failings – after all, who ever said you were supposed to be perfect?" The evidence of the research shows us that when people learn to practice self-compassion, they experience *less* depression, anxiety, stress, and shame, and *more* happiness, life-satisfaction, self-confidence, and greater physical health.

I had an opportunity to attend a one-day workshop with Dr. Neff in October 2017 and she signed my copy of her book *Self-Compassion*. This was a pivotal time for me, as I was learning how transformational this work could be and I knew that I was also interested in teaching and coaching self-compassion. I am an advocate of self-compassion because I am a living, breathing example of the positive shift that it can bring and I love that it is a practice, a tool, a strategy that you can carry with you wherever you go. As Dr. Germer says, "A moment of self-compassion can change your day. A string of such moments can change the course of your life." Being compassionate with yourself does not require any fancy equipment, you don't need to go anywhere, spend lots of money, or make an appointment with anyone other than yourself once you learn how to begin. It begins with kindness, connection, and awareness.

One of the first things that you can do to begin a self-compassion practice is learning to talk to yourself kindly. Instead of harsh words like, "Are you even trying? What is wrong with you?" I started to learn to talk to myself like I would talk to a loved one who was going through a hard time. I used words like, "I know this is hard right now. I am trying, and that's all that I can ask of myself. I am doing my best with what I have at this moment."

You can practice this kind of self-talk at the moment when you need it. You can speak these words out loud to yourself, say them silently in your head, or write them in a journal. One of the strategies in Dr. Neff's book is to write a compassionate letter to yourself as if you were writing to a good friend who needed your words of love and encouragement, but this letter is *to* you, *from* you. This has been a practice that I use often when I feel a storm of self-judgement or critical thoughts on the horizon. For example, I know that the anniversary of a trauma can be painful, especially those "firsts." Here's a letter that I wrote to myself on the eve of the one-year anniversary of my accident:

"Dear Vanessa,

"I know this feels like a hard day. It has been a difficult road. You have worked so hard. It's okay to feel sad. This has caused so many changes and so much uncertainty in your life. But you are moving forward every day. That's all you can ask of yourself. Keep going. You are doing it. This is the work. You are doing the best you can with what you have right now."

Another way to breathe life into your self-compassion practice is to remember the connection that you have to others, or *common humanity,* as Dr. Neff calls it. We are all human. We all make mistakes. It is part of our nature, and we can love ourselves through it. You can work this concept of connection into your practice of kind self-talk with words like, "Yes, you made a mistake. That did not go well. But you are human. Everyone makes mistakes. You are doing your best and it's okay to try again." Remembering that I have very human imperfections, like everyone else, helps me to stay compassionate with myself instead of jumping to harsh words and thoughts.

The third component of self-compassion is mindfulness. Mindfulness is the part of self-compassion that allows you to feel the emotions that are present, but not exaggerate or let yourself get swept away to a place of negative reactivity. Mindful self-compassion is the practice of paying attention to how you feel without harsh criticism, letting the emotions wash through you, and then picking yourself up and carrying on. In my workshops, I share an analogy about mindful self-compassion that I learned from author Glennon Doyle, and I encourage people to imagine it this way: Pain is like a traveling professor. It will come knocking on your door. Mindful self-compassion is opening the door and paying attention to what the professor is there to teach you. Feel the feelings and learn the lesson that is here for you in this moment. Once you have received the lesson, the professor is free to go.

Another important part of self-compassion is asking yourself, "What do you need?" Self-compassion is part of self-care. When you permit yourself to ask that question, I encourage you to allow all answers to flow. You might need something simple like a glass of water or some fresh air. You might need a bath or a nap. Or, you might need a friend – someone to laugh or cry with. Maybe you need to talk to a therapist or a counselor. Do you need a massage, yoga, or a Reiki treatment? Allow yourself to be curious and compassionate about what you need and then to listen to the answers.

Self-compassion is learning to set and maintain your boundaries. Boundaries refer to what is okay for you and what is not, as well as who you choose to give your time and energy to. When you are healing from a concussion and your energy is limited, it is important to learn how to communicate your boundaries. As Dr. Brené Brown teaches, "Clear is kind." Here are some examples of things you can say to protect your energy and time boundaries:

- It is not my job to take responsibility for others.
- I have a right to my own feelings.
- Nobody has to agree with me.
- I can't make it to that event this weekend.
- Yes, I'll join you, but I can only stay for an hour.
- I would love to help, but I can't right now.

Discovering what your boundaries are and what you must preserve to encourage your growth and healing, and then communicating those boundaries so that they are respected is a critical part of learning to be compassionate with yourself. As I learned from a wise friend, you can be there for the people who need you, but you get to choose who you *dance* with. When the stakes are high (which they are when you are healing), you need to show up for yourself first. It's okay to stand your sacred ground and not allow the real-estate of your head and heart to be rented out by others or by those who have not earned the right to ask this of you.

There is a myth that self-compassion is self-pity, that it is weak and soft. Let me dispel this myth. Self-compassion is often a radical choice and requires strength and courage. I have found it to be an antidote to self-pity.

Just a few weeks into the writing of this book, my mother died suddenly and unexpectedly. We were very close and she was a beautiful, connected, loving, and encouraging presence in my life. The pull to lay on the couch with the dog and a box of tissues instead of sticking to my commitment to finish this book was very real for me. But the pull to honor my mom and the work I am here to do in the world was stronger.

Here's where self-compassion became a powerful move for me and a choice. I reached for all the things I have learned. I encouraged myself with kind words, I wrote in my journal, I asked for help from friends and practitioners, I protected my time, I ate well and tried to get good sleep, I remembered that I am not alone in my grief, and I let myself feel what I was feeling. I cried when I needed to and let those tears wash through me, and I carried on, because I can choose to be compassionate with myself, even in the midst of my grief. It isn't easy and it isn't soft, but this is the yin and the yang of self-compassion. As Dr. Neff says, "We still feel pain, but we also feel the love holding the pain, and it's more bearable."

I have found self-compassion to be a very empowering tool. It is something that I am very grateful to be learning and practicing. It helps me realize that in every moment, I have a choice about how to respond to life. I am not a victim of my circumstances. I can choose to speak kindly to myself, to allow myself to feel loving and connected, to be mindful of my feelings without exaggerating them, and to set and hold my boundaries, even in the most difficult times.

8

BRAVE THE VALLEY

I love the analogy of life being a series of peaks and valleys. There is something about this analogy that feels very true and vibrant to me. The mountaintop peaks are beautiful. The views are stunning and the feeling of being on top of the world is exhilarating. Sooner or later though, there will be a walk, a fall, a stumble, and a descent into a valley, a low point. And the walk through the valley can be hard. Some days it is one foot in front of the other. After my concussion, I often found myself trudging through a valley of uncertainty and change, stumbling over the rocks in my path. The recovery and restoration that I was seeking seemed so far away. I was not the same person, but where did that leave me? Who was I now?

I have learned that trauma and transformation go hand-in-hand. It is in the valley where this transformation takes place. The valley is where things grow. It is full of life, flowing rivers, and new growth. In the midst of all the struggle I was experiencing, I found this passage from *The Women's Book of Spirit* by Sue Patton Thoele and it opened my eyes and my heart to a new perspective about the valley and the rocks that we stumble over: "Even though we can't readily see it, life teems under rocks.

Turn over a rock and notice all the little critters scurrying about, doing the business of living. So it is with us – life is teeming beneath the rocks of our day to day existence. Whether we have suffered the weight of accumulated fatigue, *or have been ripped from the very ground of our being*, it's encouraging to remember that these are fertile times for growth."

Can you find the courage to pay attention in the valley, to become curious, and to gently turn over the rocks to see what is growing underneath? The valley will come after the trauma of your experience, but it has a purpose. Find the courage and self-compassion to walk through it with open eyes and an open heart, and the valley can transform your suffering. This is a process of paying attention and reframing our challenges and how we think and talk about them.

The greatest challenges, the rocks in the river for me, felt like this:

"Will this ever get better?"

"Who am I now?"

"Are my children paying the price for my mistake, my fall?"

Let's turn over and reframe these rocks together:

Will this ever get better? It will change, it will evolve, it will be different, and maybe different isn't bad. I am still capable. I am learning to do things differently. Maybe there are treasures here that I haven't even discovered yet.

Who am I now? It's true, I am not who I was. And, I am growing, changing, and evolving. Change can be beautiful and natural, like a butterfly emerging from a cocoon.

Are my children paying the price for my mistake, my fall? Because the mother they have now is not the mother that they had. My children are watching me. Yes, they see me struggle. They see my imperfections and, in the process, they see me grow. They see my courage. They see me feel and cry and laugh and be human. Maybe they see permission to be more of themselves. They see that it is human to make mistakes. They see what self-compassion looks like. They see me learning. They see that love surrounds our family stronger than ever amid our heartbreak. They see that they will have their valleys in life, and perhaps my journey will give them the courage that they will also need one day in their own times of struggle.

This is not something you need to do by yourself. This is a good time to ask for help. I leaned on all the things I had been learning about self-care and self-compassion through this time – talking to friends and a therapist when things felt really heavy, yoga, meditation, journaling, and leaning on the team of people that I had around me through this process. They reminded me to ask for what I needed, to take care of myself, and to nourish my body, mind, and spirit.

When you are ready to reframe the challenges, here are some suggestions that can help:

- Pay attention to the words you are using. How does it feel to change "my" pain or "my" struggle to "*the* struggle."? This leaves room for the struggle or pain to be an experience or a feeling you are having, but does not insist that you grasp or hold onto it.

- Shift the words and attitude behind phrases like "I can't handle this," or "I can't do this," to "I can't handle this, *yet*." or "I am learning to do this." The words *yet* and *I am learning* provide you with the time and space you need figure it out.

- Give yourself permission to be open and curious about what insights and growth may come from this time of crisis. Try journaling with sentences like "I wonder...", and "What if...?".

- Try to imagine the challenges you are facing as clouds. Clouds move. Wounds heal. You will find clear blue sky again.

The process of turning over the rocks and looking at your challenges as something to grow from is part of healing and uncovering who you can be now, not striving or grasping to be who you were. A concussion is a brain injury. You may still have lingering symptoms. You may be a different person now in many ways. Can you give yourself permission to find the good in what is different and in what has changed? I love this wisdom from author Paulo Coelho: "Maybe the journey isn't so much about becoming anything. Maybe it's about un-becoming everything that isn't really you, so you can be who you were meant to be in the first place." This is your work. You have a choice in how to frame and speak about the transformation that is available to you after trauma. I believe that self-compassion gives you the tools, the strength, courage and power that you need to brave the valley and allow the trauma to be transformational.

The valley is here to teach you that something will grow from all you are going through. That something will be you.

9

WRITE YOUR OWN STORY

As humans, our brains have evolved massively over time. But the part of our brain that controls our most primitive survival instinct, the limbic – or "lizard brain", has not evolved since our ancient ancestors were living in a world with constant physical threats to their survival. Humans perfected a survival response - fight, flight or freeze - and adapted to live in a world of saber-tooth tigers hiding in the bushes. In fact, the effectiveness of our brain's ability to respond to stress is the reason that we as a species are still here. What does this have to do with writing stories, you ask? As human beings, our brains are also hardwired for stories with a beginning, middle and end. Stories are how we evolved in the world before we had written language. This is how we try to make sense of everything that happens to us.

Dr. Brené Brown's work in her book *Rising Strong* helped me understand the relationship between the stories that run through our thoughts and the primitive function of our lizard brain that creates these stories. In what she labels the "Rising Strong Process", Dr. Brown's research teaches us that, even though our brains have evolved in complexity and size and are capable of deep thought processes, the primitive part of our brain that is responsible for our survival still tries to run the show. Left to its own devices, it writes our stories and gives us only two options: good/bad and safe/unsafe.

Our brain will always choose a story that keeps us safe. It will always choose a story that protects us *whether the story is true or not* because that's its job – to protect us and make sure we survive. Dr. Brown calls these first stories we tell ourselves – these survival stories – our shitty first drafts, or SFDs. The SFDs that we create, whether they're true or not, often drive our thoughts which then drive our actions and behavior.

As a person who has lived through the trauma of a concussion, you may have written stories about that incident or how things are going for you through the recovery process. For the first six months after my accident, I had a story that drove my thoughts and behavior around bicycles. Bicycles were my enemy. Looking back, I now realize this was a primitive survival story. My nervous system reacted to bikes automatically, without conscious or rational thought from me. If I saw a cyclist on the road, the stress hormones would begin to race through my body and my heart would start to pound uncontrollably. Just seeing my bike or a bike helmet in the garage would cause this same reaction. To keep me safe, my brain created the shitty first draft that I should not go near a bicycle, *don't even look at them*. The primitive response in my body made me believe that this story was very real.

I am grateful that I found Dr. Brown's work during this time and that I was also referred to a therapist who knew how to help me rewrite the stories. Through our sessions, she helped me understand the neuroscience of what was happening in my brain, the survival stories that had been created, and most importantly, *that I had a choice to rewrite these stories*. There is a way to hack this process by becoming aware of the story, the shitty first draft that you are writing, and then checking the facts about what is true. Dr. Brown calls this rumbling with the truth. After the rumble, after you have gathered more true and factual information, you then have the choice to respond differently and to write a new story.

Overcoming my fear and writing a new story about bicycles was important to me because I did not want to remain a hostage to that fear my whole life. If nothing else, I wanted to be able to enjoy the simple pleasure of riding my bike through the neighborhood with my children on a warm summer day. So, one July morning, I decided that I was ready. I got clear about the story I was telling myself and I rumbled with the facts: "I *do* know how to ride a bike. This is something that I have been able to do safely for forty years. What happened to me in Italy was a freak accident. I am safe now. We have lovely bike paths throughout my neighborhood. It is a beautiful quiet morning. I want to be able to do this. I deserve to be able to do this."

It required all the courage and self-compassion that I was able to muster, and I asked my three children if they would like to go for a bike ride with me. I remember the surprise on their faces, but they agreed, and we set off together. That ride felt so brave and scary and tender and joyful. I will never forget it. I am glad that I invited my children to be with me and witness it. It empowered me to know that I could move through this process of looking at my stories, checking if they are true, and then choosing to write a new story. I did write a new story that day. I can live my life without fear in the driver's seat. As Dr.

Brown says, "Owning your story and loving yourself through this process is the bravest thing that you will ever do."

Here's another example of someone who learned to write a new story about the thoughts and behavior that she wanted to change. Liz was about a year post-concussion. Physically she was making good progress and many of her symptoms had eased, although she was not yet symptom-free. Her greatest challenge was her thoughts, her stories, and her stress about what she was capable of as she gradually returned to work and her regular activities. She struggled with thoughts like, "I am not good at this anymore. I can't do it the way I used to. I should stay home."

Now, I know this doesn't sound like life and death, but the primitive brain doesn't know the difference between the stress hormones created by our thoughts and the stress from a saber-tooth tiger. Physiologically, the thoughts feel just as real. The brain senses stress and it automatically wants to write a story that keeps us safe. Liz's shitty first draft was "I can't do this the same way I used to; therefore, it is not safe for me to even try."

But then she rumbled with her story and checked the facts. No one was expecting her to be perfect. She could take on tasks one at a time and as she gradually moved forward, she knew how to ask for help. She used this awareness to write a new story. "I am learning how to do new things in a different way. There are people here who can support me. I am capable of contributing in ways that are different, but no less effective." Liz decided to own *this* story, and it empowered her to step back into life in a way that gave her space to grow and learn, without needing to be perfect.

I encourage you to read *Rising Strong*, and if you want to dive deeper, look for a therapist or coach who is trained to facilitate this approach. Remember that asking for help if you need extra support through the process is a compassionate thing to do for yourself.

As you move forward through your healing process, I encourage you to expand your awareness of the stories that you are creating about the past, present, and what is possible for you on your road to recovery. Are the stories you are telling yourself a shitty first draft? Check in with yourself. Ask, "What is the story I am making up here? Is it true?" If the story sounds like, "I have post-concussion syndrome. This will never get better. I will always feel this way. I can't do anything that I used to do," see if you can rumble with this story.

Ask for help to gather more intel and facts. Search for resources and clinicians in your area that have up-to-date expertise and knowledge about concussions. It is never too late to seek help and treatment. Surround yourself with people who believe in the potential and possibility of your healing. Writing a new story may sound something like, "Today I have persistent symptoms. I am doing my best to heal and recover. I am learning how to take care of myself. I know that this is not a linear process and I know that complete recovery from concussions is possible."

This will give you the choice to respond and to make an informed decision about how to move forward with a story that is helpful, hopeful, and empowering for you. Remember, our stories create our thoughts which in turn drive our actions and our behavior.

You have the power to write a new ending and own your story.

10

YOU HAVE PERMISSION TO GROW

The last step in my process of reclaiming your life after a concussion is to permit yourself to feel that this can be a time of growth, change, and evolution for you that is *good*.

Nothing about this thing that happened to you may feel good, at first. It is painful. It is hard. It is confusing, not just for you, but also for your loved ones. In the first few weeks and months, your work is to rest, heal, and seek help along the way. This is a quiet time. It's a time to cultivate the soil, to plant the seeds, and to gently nourish yourself, like a garden, with just enough food, water, and sunshine. It will take time. We cannot rush or force this process. We can *nourish* it, but we cannot force it.

Then, if you pay attention, you may notice that something in this garden may begin to grow. Perhaps it's you. You may find that you are more in tune with yourself and what you need. You may grow because this concussion and this trauma you experienced has become a teacher. You have learned to listen to the clues in your body and how to take care of yourself. You grow because you honor and ask for what you need to support your healing physically, emotionally, and spiritually.

Your growth may also be an awareness that you are *uncovering* parts of yourself. My experience has been that the steps that I took to heal, the steps that I have guided you through in this book (exploring self-care, asking for and receiving help, practicing self-compassion, reframing thoughts and stories) have felt like a peeling away of layers, like an onion. I feel with each new layer that I am uncovering more of myself, who I am, what's important to me, and how I want to live my life.

You may also grow through your recovery as you get crystal clear on your values and realize what is most precious in life. A traumatic experience has the benefit of stripping away the things in our lives that are less important, as there is no extra time or energy to spend on these things. It's okay to let some things go – responsibilities, hobbies, and even relationships – to provide space for new interests, curiosities, and nourishing friendships.

Can you give yourself permission to grow through exploring your creative interests? One practice that was a creative outlet for me as I found myself changing, evolving, and *uncovering* through this process, as I mentioned in an earlier chapter, was learning to play the guitar. Another creative practice that I came to embrace was journaling. I was never fond of journaling before my concussion. Now, three years later, I have books and books filled with my thoughts, fears, learnings, and questions. I have learned so much about myself by allowing myself time and a safe place to work through my thoughts and feelings. I encourage you to nourish your creative side. Give yourself time and permission to play, explore, and wonder. If this is something that you can do with your family, what a wonderful way to allow them to grow with you!

Speaking of family, you may also notice that there has been growth and good change in your family through this process. While you never would have wished pain or struggle for them, perhaps the time you need to take for healing can open a space and create a gap for others to step in. Maybe they help out more around the house and take on tasks that they can now own. Remember the birthday party that my husband planned for our daughter? That's a perfect example. Another example of this in my house is that my three teens began to make their school lunches during the weeks after my accident. Three years later, they still own this job and I am thrilled about it!

Another example of growth in my family that began evolving through the healing process is the way we communicate with each other. As I began to learn to ask for help and *receive* it, the beautiful side-effect of this was the invitation to my loved ones to walk this road beside me by sharing our thoughts, fears, wins, and tears. We have learned that we can talk about the good things, the hard things, and everything in between. I am particularly grateful now that I invited my mom to be by my side through the whole process. We *owned* that little corner of the bookstore where we sat with our coffees every week and talked, cried, listened, and learned from each other. There is a gift in the opportunity to actively nurture and cultivate your support system through this experience. This then becomes a circle, because in the process, your family and friends will learn that there are seasons for all of us to give and receive this love and support.

In my journey over the past three years, I have met others in the concussion community who have shared a similar experience of self-discovery and growth: a musician who feels more deeply connected to his music; a painter who has uncovered tremendous talent because she sees things now that others miss; a writer whose words flow because she deeply understands what runs under the surface of things; a massage therapist who has grown her practice because she is more attuned to other people's energy and places where they feel stuck. Maybe you've discovered that you have become a better parent, partner, sister, or daughter because you know what matters now? The rest – the busyness, to-dos, should dos, and all the things that keep us separate from each other – is not what matters to you now.

Can you permit yourself to grow from this experience? In the beginning, your fears may have been about changing and you desperately just wanted to go back to being who you were, more of the same. Now that you have the steps to guide you, can you give yourself permission to grow and feel like you are uncovering more of you? This part of you was inside all along, but perhaps living under the burden of so many rules and "shoulds" that you could never hear exactly what you wanted or needed, or who you wanted to be. This experience, while we never would have wished it for you, can become a great teacher, giving you an opportunity to peel back the layers and discover things about yourself – what you might want to do, be, say, and offer to the world. I see hope and power in this for you.

11

THE HURDLES YOU WILL FACE

As we both know, the path to feeling healthy and whole again and like you are back on your feet and able to reclaim your life is a winding road. There are good days and challenging days, and symptoms that may persist or return even when you thought you finally had it all together.

One hurdle to overcome is a belief that things must be tidy and perfect before you can *live again*. You can choose to leap over this hurdle if you decide that you can love yourself through both kinds of days, the good days and the bad ones. The days when you feel on top of the world again and the days that remind you that the valley is hard. Author Glennon Doyle sums this up perfectly when she says, "Life is brutal and life is beautiful. Brutiful, I call it. Life's brutal and beautiful are woven together so tightly that they are inseparable. We must embrace both or neither." Can you embrace your brutiful life? The days that feel easy and the days that everything feels so hard? You have learned how to do this through the steps in this book.

There is another hurdle that you will need to gather the courage to cross – *"If you fight for your limitations, you get to keep them."*

I learned this from renowned brain science expert Jim Kwik. You may bump up against this hurdle often, and it is one of the reasons why I wrote this book. When I realized that I was one of the thirty to thirty-five percent of people who deal with lingering post-concussion symptoms, I looked for community and support in many places, but noticed that some people had a tendency to stay stuck. They put a great deal of their precious energy into fighting for their limitations – focusing on the negative.

We definitely need to acknowledge and face the difficulties that come with a concussion, but I was also seeking current information and resources to help me feel empowered and hopeful. I was seeking a community that would focus on potential and possibility, not limitations. If this resonates with you, I encourage you to check out MollyParkerPT on social media. Molly's content was the first online experience I had that blended up-to-date expertise with a realistic but positive focus on healing and useful information. Molly is a doctor of physical therapy and is also straddling the post-concussion world as a patient. So, check in with yourself to ask where you might be fighting for your limitations. It's natural for us, as humans, to lean to a negativity bias, but the words that we use do affect how we feel. If you are fighting for your limitations, you might miss the opportunity to see all the ways you are growing and evolving.

Another hurdle that you might have to cross as you work to get back on your feet is a thought that your loved ones don't want you to change and grow. Can we rumble with that story and ask, "is it true?". We are social beings and our brains are wired with ancient survival stories that if we change and get kicked out of the tribe, we will die. I had to battle this hurdle too, but my experience through this journey is that my friends and family want good things for me. When they see that I am growing and evolving, they are usually happy for me and in many cases, growing *with* me. And the ones that aren't? I let them go, knowing that they are not meant for me anymore. All that said, I do realize that while this is my experience, yours may be very different. I have listened to stories from people I have met in the concussion community whose relationships came apart, rather than together, during this experience. I believe that each story, each family and the healing journey for each of us is unique. I hold a tender space for your story whether it is similar to mine in how you were loved and supported, or whether it was very different.

There will be times when you feel completely dialed-in to your self-care routine – your nutrition, yoga, and exercise game is strong, and then something happens and you want nothing but comfort food, the couch, and Netflix. You will go through these ups and downs. God knows, I certainly have. I try to navigate this hurdle with compassion for myself. You're the only one who knows the answer to "What do I need right now?" Sometimes, the answer is to take a compassionate break.

When your self-care slips for a prolonged period though, try to practice kind self-talk. *You are human. It's normal to struggle sometimes. What do you need that will help you get back to feeling good?* Pay attention to the emotions behind the slip. For example, if you're reaching for food to numb how you're feeling you can ask, "Is there something else that can help me move through this emotion?" Perhaps in that moment a warm bath, or talking to a friend will fill that need? Remember that self-compassion isn't about being soft. It's about talking to yourself like someone you love, and sometimes the most loving answer to "What do I need right now?" is a gentle reminder to *Get up. Move your body. Drink a glass of water. Eat something that will nourish you.*

You do not have to be who you were. Remember that you have the power to write your own story. Are you stuck on the hurdle that your only option for recovery is the striving to get back to "normal," to your old self? Is this the only outcome you will accept? If so, I encourage you to ask yourself, "What if? What if it was okay to evolve, grow, change, and want different things? What if there is more? What if, in all the ways that I am now different and new, I am also more of myself?" There is an opening here, an opportunity for you to write a new story, to own this story and write your ending if you have the courage to leap clear over the hurdle that says you are now less than you were.

We all face challenges in life, and a post-concussion journey is no different. As you come to these hurdles it helps to remember that since childhood you have encountered challenges and had to learn new things. We learn by trying, and failure is just a try that hasn't worked yet. These hurdles – that conditions must be perfect for you to *live* your life, fighting for your limitations, resisting growth and grasping for your "old self," and fear that people won't accept a "new you," – can be faced and overcome. It is actually this adversity that helps us become resilient.

This quote by Napoleon Hill frames adversity and resilience for us: "The strongest oak tree of the forest is not the one that is protected from the storm and hidden from the sun. It's the one that stands in the open where it is compelled to struggle for its existence against the winds and the rain and the scorching sun." Facing your hurdles and trying to cross them one day at a time will help your roots grow deep and resilient.

12

MY WISH FOR YOU

t took me many, many months to pick up the pieces of my life after my concussion. Even when I had a handle on most of my physical symptoms, anything that lingered, even if it was mild, triggered thoughts that I had changed, I was different, I was less than, I had lost a part of me. The real work in this process was figuring out how to shift my thoughts so that I could accept these symptoms as a physical reality at that moment. But my thoughts were a choice that I was making. I needed to learn to *choose* different thoughts and write different stories. It takes awareness and courage to realize that this is what you need and to do this work.

I hope that the steps in this book can be a guide for you to do this work, reclaim your life, and continue your healing journey confident that you have someone to guide you forward in how you love and care for yourself. You have learned how to practice good self-care, how to ask for help when you need it, how to receive that help, and how to talk to yourself like you talk to a loved one. You know that the love you give is *for you too,* so that on the hard days when you're walking through the valley, you can allow yourself to receive and feel that love. You have learned how to reframe your challenges and your "rocks," and how to write a brave ending to your story, one that is hopeful, positive, and empowering. Finally, you know that you have permission to be even more than you were before. Although no one would have wished this for you, you have permission to grow and change from it. Life is happening for you.

I wish for you to begin to breathe self-compassion into your body, your bones, and your cells. It is not easy. It is not soft. It is asking for what you need. It is paying attention to how you feel. It is giving yourself time to be still and quiet and to listen. It is learning from your pain, not wallowing in it. It is allowing yourself to change and evolve. It is what brings you joy now and what makes you feel alive. It is allowing yourself to uncover and become someone new. It is having the courage to use your voice and to speak your truth. Self-compassion is learning how to nourish your heart, your mind, and your body with food, movement, creativity, curiosity, play, and connection to others. It is believing, speaking, and choosing as if the love you give is for you too. It is receiving the love and support that others offer you because this is the garden that you have cultivated your whole life. If you haven't sown those seeds, then it is never too late to start.

I know this to be true – you are loved exactly as you are. This was the greatest lesson of my fall and concussion. I am loved. Not because of what I do, but just because I am. My greatest failure taught me the greatest lesson of my life. I want you to know it too. You are worthy. Especially in those moments that feel like the biggest mistakes, falls, and failures. Those are the moments when you are most loved and held. This understanding of grace came to me through being cracked open, head and heart. It is my wish for you that your concussion, your heartbreak, and your loss might open you up as well to the life and love that is happening for you.

ACKNOWLEDGMENTS

To my husband Oliver – when I decided that it was time for me to write this book, you offered me your full support and said, "Let's clear the decks." It was your intention for me to write this book with ease and joy. Two weeks after I said an enthusiastic "yes!" to the Author Incubator, my mom passed away very suddenly and a tsunami of grief swept into our lives. Thank you for being both my rock and my soft place, again. Although you could not take away this pain, I know you shouldered it with me. You calmly created the space in my life and in our home that I needed, so that I could be the person who finished anyway, with all the ease and joy that you could help me find. *I love you.*

To our extraordinary children Galen, Noah, and Madeleine – you are the greatest source of joy, fun, love, and laughter in my life. Thank you for being proud, patient and encouraging cheerleaders for me through this process. When the big things feel out of control, you three remind me what matters most. There is more fun in store for W5! I promise.

To Rebecca, Denise, Tina, Brenda, Renee, Lianne, Karen S., and my entire circle of friends – thank you for the hugs, encouraging words, check-ins, coffee dates, meals shared, laughter, tissues, and help in *all* the ways you offer it. I am grateful for each one of you and the precious gifts that you each have and share so freely with me.

To my healers and helpers, especially Mark and Karen L. – you are the bridge that helps me hear what my body, mind, and spirit want me to know. Thank you for helping me hear and trust my voice.

Dr. Angela, Ramses, Emily, and the team at the Author Incubator – thank you for your coaching and support and for helping me free my inner author. Thank you for holding space for nothing but my success and for helping me get over the finish line.

Finally, a story from the dedication in this book that I want to share with you about my parents – my father, Terry, passed away from cancer when I was eighteen. He was a force of nature and had a personality that was larger than life. He loved us fiercely, and I knew it. We sang a hymn called "On Eagle's Wings" at his funeral and we had those words engraved on his headstone.

My mother, Peggy, passed away, very suddenly and unexpectedly, as I began writing this book in the fall of 2019. She was my best friend, my confidante, my North Star. It felt to me like the earth shifted on its axis when she died.

At her funeral in St. George's Anglican Church in Guelph, Ontario, my brother and I spoke words to honor her, remember her, and comfort our grieving family and friends. As I stood at the front of the church that day, mustering the courage to speak about her legacy of love, I realized that my hand was holding on tight to the wing of a golden eagle, the sculpture that stands majestically at the St. George's pulpit. On one of the most difficult days of my life, I found an eagle's wing beside me, to raise me up and carry me through.

THANK YOU

Thank you so much for reading *Bounce Back: The Guide to Reclaiming Your Life After a Concussion.* Since you've finished reading, I know that you are on the path to bouncing back after the frustration, loss, and change a concussion can bring. This can be a long and difficult process for some people and I want to support you as much as possible.

If you are interested in a one-on-one phone call with me to learn more about how you can bounce back after a concussion, email me at bounceback@woodburn.ca to schedule a free thirty-minute phone consultation to share your story, to ask questions and learn about the steps I teach – the steps that I learned as I healed from a concussion in 2016.

I look forward to hearing from you!

ABOUT THE AUTHOR

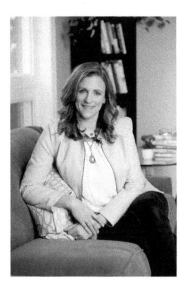

Vanessa Woodburn is a certified health coach, educator and author. Her work is centered around resilience, self-compassion, and helping people bounce back after concussion and setback - mind, body, and spirit. Vanessa has successfully navigated this path herself and is the perfect person to guide others through this experience. Her passion for healing shines through in her workshops, talks, and coaching. Vanessa began her career as a special education teacher, but changed tracks a few years later.

She graduated from the Institute for Integrative Nutrition™ as a Health Coach in 2017. Vanessa's calling to coach people through setbacks led her to pursue further education in cultivating compassion through the Compassion Institute and Self-Compassion workshops with Dr. Kristin Neff. She weaves her years of experience in education, wellness, health, resilience, and compassion into her coaching and talks. Vanessa lives in Mississauga, Ontario, with her husband Oliver and three teens. She enjoys relaxing at the family cottage, listening to music, reading and traveling adventures with her husband and kids.